The Honey Revolution

(Abridged)

The Honey Revolution

Restoring the Health of Future Generations
(Abridged)

Ron Fessenden, MD, MPH
Mike McInnes, MRPS

WorldClassEmprise, LLC
Colorado Springs, Colorado

© 2010 Ron Fessenden and Mike McInnes. Printed and bound in the United States of America. All rights reserved. No part of this book may be reproduced or transmitted in any form or by any means, electronic or mechanical, including photocopying, recording, or by an information storage and retrieval system—except by a reviewer, who may quote brief passages in a review to be printed in a magazine, newspaper, or on the web—without permission in writing from the publisher. For information, please contact WorldClassEmprise, LLC, 24 Luxury Lane, Colorado Springs, CO 80921; 719-481-1411.

The publisher makes no representation, express or implied, regarding the accuracy of the information contained in this work, and legal responsibility or liability cannot be accepted by the authors or the publisher for any errors or omissions that may be made or for any loss, damage, injury, or problems suffered or in any way arising from following the nutritional advice offered in these pages.

First printing 2010

ISBN: 978-0-9792162-0-6
LCCN: 2010938818

ATTENTION CORPORATIONS, UNIVERSITIES, COLLEGES, AND PROFESSIONAL ORGANIZATIONS: Discounts are available on bulk purchases of this book for educational or gift purposes, or as premiums for increasing magazine subscriptions or renewals. Special edition books or book excerpts can also be created to fit specific needs. For information, please contact WorldClassEmprise, LLC, 24 Luxury Lane, Colorado Springs, CO 80921; 719-481-1411.

www.worldclassemprise.com

CONTENTS

Note to the Reader 7

**The Honey Revolution:
Changing the Way We Think About Honey** 9

Health Benefits of Consuming Honey 11

Honey: More Than Just a Sweetener 15

    Your Dietary Shift Is Showing 17

    Differentiating Honey from Other Sweeteners 20

    It's Counterintuitive but True:
    How Honey Regulates Blood Sugar 25

    Becky and Reactive Hypoglycemia 26

    Honey Versus Artificial Sweeteners 27

    The Dieter's Dilemma and Artificial Sweeteners 29

Honey: Nature's Amazing Medicine 31

    Honey and Sleep 31

    Liver Glycogen Depletion Rate in Grams Versus Time . 34

    Honey for Depression 35

    Honey for Diabetes 36

    Duane's Diabetes and Honey Story 37

    Honey for Gastrointestinal Health 39

    Honey for the Heart 40

    Honey for the Immune System 40

    Honey for Melatonin and the Mind 41

    Honey for Menopause and Infertility 41

    Honey for Sleep Disorders 42

    Honey for Thyroid Conditions 43

    Honey and Dreams 43

    Honey and Alzheimer's Disease 44

    Honey and Aging 46

    Directives for Better Health 47

Honey: The Superfuel for Exercise 49

    The Five Critical Times for Fueling for Exercise 50

    Don't Be Confused About Energy 51

    Ten Basic Facts for Exercise Fueling 52

Honey: The All-Star Superfood 55

    Another "Believer" Joined the Revolution 55

    How Much Honey Is Enough 57

Frequently Asked Questions 59

References 69

About the Authors 71

NOTE TO THE READER

ONE MIGHT CONCLUDE after a casual reading of the table of contents or a brief perusal of this short book that honey is being presented as a "cure" for many diseases and conditions. Such is not the case. Honey is a healthful food to be sure, but it cannot reverse what months and years of dietary indiscretions, lifestyle choices, and/or genetics have caused. Regular honey consumption at bedtime, for example, will result in improved sleep patterns and reduced nighttime metabolic stress almost immediately for most individuals. However, many disease processes as well as their ultimate prognoses may be irreversible.

The information provided in this book is not intended to be a substitute for the advice and counsel of your personal physician. Suggestions regarding the use of honey are recommendations, not prescriptions or medical guidelines for self-treatment, and should not be substituted for any treatment recommendations prescribed by your physician. While the recommendations are appropriate and risk free for most people, each individual has differing requirements and/or responses to dietary recommendations based on one's complete medical profile. The reader should also note that reductions in risks for any disease or condition are determined across large populations and do not necessarily apply to each individual within that population.

Finally, throughout the pages of this book, short stories of real people appear in shaded text, though the names have been changed. Some stories are told as if only one individual is sharing his/her experience, but the story is often representative of multiple individuals' stories, all sharing the same facts.

The Honey Revolution: Changing the Way We Think About Honey

WEBSTER'S ONLINE DICTIONARY defines "revolution" as "a fundamental change in the way of thinking about or visualizing something: a change of paradigm. . . ." That is exactly why this short book was written—to help change the way we think about honey. This miraculous food is often referred to as "nature's sweetener," but categorizing honey as a sweetener communicates a lesser truth about honey. Beyond its sweetness, honey is a natural food that contains many health-promoting properties. It is a superfood—a revolutionary food—bringing many health benefits to those who consume it regularly.

Health Benefits of Consuming Honey

It is important to differentiate between a health *benefit* and a health *claim*! The difference is not just semantics. Health claims are typically validated by well-controlled, double-blind studies conducted with large population or study groups. The results are usually only applicable for that study population given the strict protocols by which the research is conducted. Many times, health claims validated by large research studies are ignored or overlooked. For example, there are numerous population studies that link consumption of HFCS (high-fructose corn syrup) to obesity, childhood obesity, and diabetes. The same can be said of sucrose (or table sugar), yet the FDA and most medical organizations remain silent.

Health benefits are no less significant even though they may not have the weight of an FDA-approved health claim. For example, most readers understand that foods containing antioxidants are good for one's health. That is a health benefit statement based on the general knowledge of the role of antioxidants in the body. Likewise, general knowledge of human physiology, as well as information gained from several smaller research studies (both human and animal), allows us to underscore the many health benefits available from consuming honey. For example, the consumption of 3 to 5 tablespoons of honey a day, while at the same time reducing consumption of sucrose and HFCS, can result in the following health benefits: a more regulated metabolism, stabilized blood sugar levels, reduction in HbA1c (glycated hemoglobin in the blood) and triglyceride levels (energy that stores fat in the body), and a lowered risk for diseases associated with the metabolic syndrome.[1]

A health benefit is simply something that improves or is of benefit to your general health. No claims are to be inferred as to when, to what degree, or how broadly these benefits apply across a large population. And many health benefits work to prevent other diseases or conditions. Most importantly, the health benefits derived from consuming honey *come at no risk and with no negative health consequences.*

Other health benefit statements regarding honey appear throughout this book. These statements are based on facts derived from many sources, including the following:

1. Animal studies that show lowered blood sugar levels, increased memory, and decreased anxiety from consuming honey versus glucose or artificial sweeteners

---

[1] The metabolic syndrome includes the following diseases and conditions: adult and childhood obesity, type 2 diabetes, cardiovascular disease, arrhythmia, hypertension, stroke, osteoporosis, hypothyroidism, depression, Alzheimer's disease, dementia, and sleep disorders.

2. Observational studies that simply report measurable differences following consumption of honey versus glucose or sucrose (e.g., a Honey Tolerance Test versus a Glucose Tolerance Test [GTT])

3. Accepted knowledge of human physiology such as the benefits of restorative sleep and the reduction of metabolic stress that come from stocking the liver glycogen store (both of which can be enhanced by the consumption of a tablespoon or two of honey before bedtime)

4. "Connecting the dots" in which physiologic and metabolic principles are linked to certain outcomes (e.g., honey promotes restorative sleep, which will in turn reduce the risk of hypertension and many conditions associated with the metabolic syndrome)

Many of the health benefit statements made in this book will seem outrageous to some. Where are the references? Where is the proof? Believe us, the evidence is extensive. But because this is an abridged version intended to present summaries rather than details, all the references have been omitted. The skeptical reader is invited to review the full version of *The Honey Revolution* and a second book by the authors to be published in 2010 entitled *Smart Sleep: How to Sleep Your Way to Better Health (with Honey)*. These unabridged editions contain over 300 references and endnotes compiled from the world's literature that support the statements made in this short book.

Following are eight of the most important health benefits derived by consuming honey on a regular basis:

1. Honey consumption results in a lower insulin response than that produced by similar amounts of sucrose or

HFCS, and its regular consumption will result in less weight gain and a lowered risk for diabetes.

2. Unlike eating HFCS, eating honey does not result in elevated triglycerides, and the fructose in honey actually protects against triglyceride formation.

3. Honey promotes restorative sleep, and restorative sleep reduces risk for hypertension.

4. Honey lowers levels of HCY (homocysteine), an amino acid involved in cellular metabolism and the manufacture of proteins. Elevated HCY levels are responsible for about 10 percent of the coronary deaths each year.

5. By stabilizing blood sugar levels, honey improves memory and cognitive ability.

6. Honey has a direct effect on lowering cortisol levels through its promotion of liver glycogen formation and lowering of blood sugar. Depression and anxiety are associated with elevated cortisol levels.

7. Honey lowers cancer risks by reducing obesity. Obesity is directly responsible for over 100,000 cancer deaths in the Unites States per year.

8. The fructose from honey restores NAD, the liver enzyme responsible for the detoxification of alcohol.

Honey: More Than Just a Sweetener

"Conventional wisdom" among physicians, nutritionists, dietitians, and other health professionals is that honey is only a sugar and needs to be considered as such in relation to blood sugar control. The great majority of health professionals represent this school of thought and practice. Fortunately for us all, conventional wisdom is being overturned by contemporary science and reinforced by anecdotal evidence.

Over the past several months, we have received several testimonials from individuals who have started consuming honey in an attempt to control their blood sugar and "treat" their diabetes. One ninety-year-old pastor from California tracked his blood sugar levels faithfully every day for one month before starting to consume a tablespoon of honey at bedtime. His daily blood sugar readings averaged 148 milligrams percent. In the first month after beginning his "honey therapy," his blood sugar levels averaged 138 milligrams percent; the second month, they dropped to an average of 110, where they remained for an additional six months. Others have reported similar amazing results that have confounded their physicians. When offering the explanation that consuming honey, usually at bedtime, is the reason blood sugar levels have stabilized and their HbA1c levels have come down, the disbelieving physician often responds by saying, "That can't be so. Honey is only a sugar!"

The physician is speaking the truth as far as he/she understands it. Honey is composed of two principle sugars, glucose and fructose, just the same as HFCS and sucrose. The ratio of fructose to glucose in all three sweeteners is nearly the same (one to one, or close to it). However, the physician's knowledge of honey and its effects on human metabolism is, unfortunately, shallow and misinformed.

What makes honey unique? On what basis can one distinguish honey from its "competitors"? The answers to these questions are given in detail in the following pages.

First, let's take a step back and discover the origins of this sweet natural food given to us by the Creator. The process of creating honey begins as photons from the sun stimulate photosynthesis by bombarding chloroplasts in plants. These plants then mature, flower, and produce nectar, a sweet combination of sucrose and glucose in differing ratios.

Next comes the honeybee. The honeybee gathers nectar from a diversity of floral sources, preferring nectar that contains a mixture of glucose and sucrose rather than one predominating in either sugar. Enzymes in the honeybee's honey sac (a specialized collecting chamber in the bee for storage of foraged nectar and pollen) degrade or split the sucrose into fructose and glucose, producing a blend containing a nearly equal ratio of both sugars—nature's perfect ratio required for the formation of liver glycogen, which is the primary fuel for the brain.

This conversion by the honeybee of sucrose to glucose and fructose comes at a high energy toll, a fact that argues against some chance occurrence or metabolic accident and argues for intentional design by the Creator. It was clearly in the Creator's plan to provide us with this wonderful, miraculous food—the food that we call *honey*.

Your Dietary Shift Is Showing

The significance of honey in nutritional considerations might be lost completely if it were not for a not-so-subtle event that has been occurring over the past forty years in the United States —an event characterized by the shift away from fats in our diet to a predominance of carbohydrates. This dietary shift has produced results that we can all see firsthand, whether in our daily glances in the mirror or while "people gazing" wherever we may be.

Since the 1970s, when "new conventional wisdom" began to emphasize an avoidance of saturated fats, a tragic result of epidemic proportions has occurred. Two out of three individuals are now overweight or obese in the United States, which includes 20 percent of children under the age of eighteen. Over 24 million U.S. citizens have diabetes (nearly 10 percent), and a staggering 57 million are pre-diabetic. The economic costs are enormous, now approaching $200 billion annually for diabetes alone.

The World Health Organization and other public health advisory groups recommend that no more than 40 percent of our daily caloric intake should come from carbohydrates. No more than 10 percent of our total calorie intake each day should come from simple sugars (sucrose, glucose, fructose, lactose). Unfortunately, 60 to 80 percent (and sometimes more) of our current daily intake comes from carbohydrates—nearly double the recommended amount.

Of course there are causes for this epidemic "shift" other than just the increased consumption of carbohydrates. Sedentary lifestyles, lack of exercise, dependence on technology, reduction in physical labor, genetics—all can be blamed. But the preponderance of evidence relating to our weighty health problem corresponds, not so coincidently, to this marked shift in the percentage of carbohydrates being consumed in our diets each day, especially sugar and HFCS.

A major irony in this dietary shift is that while being "fat" is epidemic, fats are not the problem! What started in the 1960s as the "dietary fat hypothesis" has resulted in the largest public health issue of this new century. In the late 1940s, the Framingham Heart Study in Massachusetts began collecting data on 8000 men. By the mid 1960s, it appeared that saturated fats in the diet were apparently associated with an increased incidence of cardiovascular disease (heart attacks and strokes). From this apparent association came the widely accepted mantra "beware of saturated fats," and over the next two decades "low-fat everything" became the accepted norm!

It was not until 1992 that Dr. William Castelli, the original director of the Framingham Study, blew the whistle on this myth that had by that time become an accepted fact for nearly everyone. In an article published in the *Archives of Internal Medicine* that year, Dr. Castelli stated, "the people with the lowest serum cholesterol were the ones who ate the most saturated fat and cholesterol, and took in the most calories." So much for this indictment of dietary fats!

Another irony in this dietary shift is that low-fat foods are actually more problematic, contributing to the fat epidemic rather than reducing it. One critical observation is that it didn't take long for processed food manufacturers to discover just how to make low-fat foods taste good: just add sugar or HFCS. So much sugar and HFCS has been added and consumed during the age of processed foods that the annual per capita consumption of these sweeteners now approaches 160 pounds—over 3 pounds per week!

The unheralded truth about human metabolism is that one does not get fat by eating fat. *One gets fat by eating too much sugar!* Beware of products that market "low-fat" and "healthy" on the packaging. Check the label for sugar or HFCS content and decide for yourself if "low-fat" is worth the risk.

One product in particular that illustrates this marketing sleight of hand is "low-fat" or "light" yogurt. Food manufacturers have flooded the market with these products, which now occupy several shelves of the supermarket coolers. The irony is that relatively small amounts of harmless milk fats are removed and excessive quantities of sugar or HFCS or both are dumped in. Then, supported by huge advertising budgets, the product is promoted as a healthy option. The reality is that regular yogurt sweetened with a small amount of honey is much better for you.

The past forty years have witnessed a constant rise in the amount of sugar and HFCS consumed (with the exception of the past three years, during which the consumption has leveled out somewhat). *Three pounds a week* for every man, woman, child, and infant in the United States each year may not seem like a lot, but compare that to the annual per capita consumption of other "staples" such as french fries (55 pounds), chocolate (over 12 pounds), garlic (3.5 pounds), peanut butter (3 pounds), and honey (only 1 pound).

In March 2010, the American Heart Association recommended that consumption guidelines for sugars be added to food products. Their benchmark was 25 grams per day for women and 37.5 grams for men. That amount doesn't include the natural sugars that are found in fruits, vegetables, and milk products. Compare this AHA benchmark with the approximately 200 grams per capita of sugar and HFCS currently consumed daily. Is there any wonder why we are a generation of fat people?

Differentiating Honey from Other Sweeteners

To better appreciate the role of honey as a healthful food, it is first helpful to look at the sweeteners to which honey is frequently compared. *Sucrose*, or common table sugar, is a simple sugar—a disaccharide made up of equal parts of two sugars, glucose and fructose. When ingested, an enzyme in the gut breaks the bond holding the fructose and glucose molecules together, allowing them to pass easily into the blood stream. The circulating blood then delivers the fructose and glucose to the liver and on to other cells of the body.

Glucose can be used for energy by nearly every cell in the body while fructose can only be metabolized in the liver. Excess glucose is stored as glycogen in muscle cells or fat in either muscle cells or adipose (fatty) tissue around the abdominal organs.

Excessive consumption of sucrose is associated with obesity; diabetes; insulin resistance; and the metabolic syndrome and its associated conditions, including hypertension, elevated blood lipids, cardiovascular disease, osteoporosis, some forms of cancer, polycystic ovarian disease, Alzheimer's disease, and more. It has even been said that if FDA approval of sugar as a food additive were to be requested today, it would not be given!

HFCS is made from cornstarch, which is mostly glucose. Enzymatic action catalyzed by hydrochloric acid produces fructose from the glucose. Once the solution reaches a concentration of 90 percent fructose, glucose is added back in to arrive at the ratios commonly used in food manufacturing and processing today—55:45 or 42:58 of fructose to glucose.

Of the sweeteners used in foods and drinks in the United States today, HFCS represents about 40 percent. Until recently, 100 percent of the soft drinks bottled here used HFCS as the primary sweetener. Within the past few months, the negative publicity surrounding HFCS has forced bottling companies to begin using sugar again. The same is also occurring in food processing, with food manufacturers shifting toward putting "Contains no HFCS" on their package labels. What is not being told, however, is that *excessive HFCS consumption has just the same effects in the body as does excessive sugar consumption*. A conservative estimate of HFCS consumption indicates that *the daily average for all Americans aged two and above is 330 grams (0.73 pounds), or 1320 calories, from HFCS* alone!

What is the problem with sugar and HFCS? Don't they have similar fructose to glucose ratios and the same caloric density as honey? That's the argument used by the Corn

Refiners Association on their website. The challenge for the honey industry and for those who drive public health policy is to *differentiate* honey from other sweeteners. As the demand for and consumption of other sweeteners declines commensurate with an increase in information as to the disastrous health effects of these sweeteners, the consumption of honey will also decrease unless we educate and inform. On the surface, this is a formidable challenge.

When comparing the fructose and glucose content alone, there is little difference between honey, sucrose, and HFCS. However, once one gets past the initial similarities, honey is a unique natural food that can be differentiated in several ways.

1. Honey contains more than 180 different substances that have been isolated from various honey varietals. These include 5 enzymes, 6 different vitamins, 8 distinctive lipids, 12 minerals, 17 trace elements, 18 different acids, 18 amino acids (proteins), 18 bioflavonoids (also known as antioxidants), and 26 aroma compounds. In this regard, *honey is more like a fruit than a sugar.* Sucrose and HFCS are much simpler compounds by comparison, made up primarily of glucose and fructose.

2. Honey is metabolized, partitioned, and stored in the body differently than sucrose or HFCS. The key to understanding this difference requires an understanding of how the body metabolizes and stores glucose. The body has two primary storage areas for glucose: muscle tissue and the liver. These tissues store glucose as glycogen, which is simply multiple molecules of glucose joined together by an easily reducible bond. Muscle tissue can store about 800 to 1000 grams of glycogen. The liver can only store about 80 to 100 grams—only one-tenth as much. Whereas glucose can enter most cells in the body

freely, the liver cells use fructose to facilitate the entry of glucose into the liver cell, where it can be converted to glycogen and stored. It is the fructose molecule that unlocks or releases glucokinase from the liver cell nucleus. Glucokinase is the enzyme necessary for the liver cell to create glycogen from glucose. A small dose of honey (1 to 2 tablespoons, or about 20 to 40 grams), with its small fructose portion, is ideal for replenishing liver glycogen levels. Liver glycogen is the primary fuel reserve for the brain, and *honey ingestion results in liver glycogen formation directly.*

3. Sucrose or HFCS in the amounts typically ingested in the average diet do not form liver glycogen directly. Rather, the large glucose load contained in these sugars bypasses the liver and triggers a massive insulin response, driving circulating glucose into muscle and fat cells, where it is used for energy or is more likely stored as fat. *The excessive sucrose and HFCS ingestion of the modern diet results in fat storage; the same is not true of honey consumed in moderation.*

4. The typical load of fructose (contained in sucrose or HFCS) consumed by the average person is simply overwhelming to the liver, which is the only organ that can metabolize fructose. The liver stops everything else that it is doing, including the production of glycogen, to metabolize the fructose. It does this by converting the fructose into trioses, or three-carbon molecules, which enter the fatty acid cycle to form triglycerides and then get stored as fat. *Excessive fructose ingestion results in fat formation and storage—a problem that does not occur when small amounts of fructose (as found in honey) are consumed.*

It is at this point in the narrative that someone usually asks, "What if a person consumed the same amount of honey daily as he/she would consume of sucrose and HFCS on average in the modern daily diet? Wouldn't the results be the same, as they are essentially the same sugars?" The answer lies in the book of Wisdom in the Old Testament (Proverbs 25:16 [NIV]): "If you find honey, eat just enough—too much of it, and you will vomit." It is safe to conclude without personal experimentation that this is a true statement: the body naturally purges itself of excess levels of honey (unlike the unhealthy absorption/processing of excess levels of simple sugars like sucrose and HFCS).

An additional differentiation of honey and glucose is possible from direct observation and recording of measurable events in the body following ingestion of equal quantities of these foods. A Honey Tolerance Test (similar to the Glucose Tolerance Test, or GTT) is a good illustration. A dose of honey is ingested and blood sugar levels are measured at several intervals following administration; the same is done with glucose at a separate time. When compared to the glucose tests, results from the honey tests at 60 and 90 minutes after consumption show a 20 and 40 milligrams percent lower blood sugar level respectively. (Note: milligrams percent, or mg%, measures the number of milligrams of a given chemical in 100 milliliters of blood.)

Here are a few more observations that serve to differentiate honey from sucrose or HFCS:

1. **Honey consumption stabilizes blood sugar levels.** The glucose from honey enters the liver directly to form liver glycogen. As glucose is removed from the blood, hyperglycemia (high blood sugar) is prevented and blood sugar levels are maintained within a normal range.

2. **Honey consumption prevents hypoglycemia.** The direct formation of liver glycogen from honey helps to maintain adequate liver glycogen levels and prevents hypoglycemia, especially during sleep and exercise.

3. **Honey consumption reduces intracellular oxidative stress**, which is the underlying cause of many diseases and conditions associated with the metabolic syndrome and diseases of aging. Hyperglycemia is the primary cause of intracellular oxidative stress and can be prevented by stabilizing blood sugar levels with the help of honey.

4. **Honey consumption reduces metabolic stress.** This is an example of what may be called "connecting the dots" of health benefits. Metabolic stress occurs when the brain is in danger of running out of fuel, as during exercise and during the night fast. Therefore, honey consumption before a workout or before bedtime ensures an adequate store of liver glycogen for the brain and prevents or reduces the release of stress hormones (adrenalin and cortisol) from the adrenal glands.

5. **Honey consumption allows recovery sleep to proceed uninterrupted** by reducing or preventing the occurrence of metabolic stress during the early morning hours (an event triggered by the hungry brain in search of fuel). Restoration of mind and body can then occur normally during the night hours.

It's Counterintuitive but True: How Honey Regulates Blood Sugar

The fact that honey regulates blood sugar seems counterintuitive—sort of like eating bacon to lower your cholesterol. The secret of honey's ability to regulate blood sugar lies in its balance of fructose and glucose. The fructose in honey allows the glucose portion to be taken in by the liver to form glycogen. Glucose is thus removed from circulation and blood sugar levels are lowered. *Honey consumed regularly in small doses throughout the day prevents hyperglycemia.*

The fact that honey consumption results in the direct formation of liver glycogen rather than in causing an elevation of blood sugar serves several purposes. A replete liver glycogen store provides the body with immediate access to glucose at any time when blood sugar levels are low, such as during exercise or while sleeping, or in situations known as reactive hypoglycemia. Liver glycogen fuels the brain at times when it is most at risk of running out of fuel, such as during exercise and during the night fast. At all times, the liver releases its glycogen store on demand to share with all other organs in the body. *Thus, honey prevents hypoglycemia through its direct formation of liver glycogen and its release from the liver on demand.*

Becky and Reactive Hypoglycemia

Becky had a successful career as an administrative assistant for a corporate VP for more than thirty years. Her life was packed with episodic stress on the job that began most mornings at 6:00 AM and lasted into the evening hours, five to six days a week. Her eating patterns were as consistent as work demands allowed, yet frequently she suffered from bouts of shakiness, lightheadedness, nausea, and diminished concentration. Her early morning wake-ups were especially difficult and symptomatic. Occasionally work hours were punctuated with bouts of shakiness and nausea. Her self-diagnosis was "low blood sugar," and her solution was to grab a cup of coffee and a chocolate donut to get her through. In a matter of minutes, her symptoms were relieved only to return again in a couple of hours.

A friend suggested that she try a tablespoon of honey at bedtime. It seemed crazy, but she took the advice. In a matter of days, she began to notice significant changes. She was no longer awakened with the intense nausea, shakiness, and malaise. She now felt like eating a good breakfast and seemed to get through the day to an early lunch without experiencing any symptoms. She also began taking "honey sticks" to work for use when the workload kept her at her desk.

In less than a few weeks, she pronounced herself "cured" and symptom free, thanks to a bit of honey before bedtime. When she retired in the fall of 2008, Becky remarked that she owed her longevity on the job to honey!

Honey Versus Artificial Sweeteners

Many who are concerned about their weight or who are diabetic or pre-diabetic use artificial sweeteners almost exclusively, as most physicians recommend this substitution to them. Those who are disciplined about following this advice often become frustrated with their inability to lose weight, however. Some even buy "sugar-free" honey from one of the big box stores thinking that it is a good substitute for sugar! Many find that their blood sugar levels continue to swing widely throughout the day and are elevated in the early morning hours in spite of having had nothing to eat since the night before.

The problem with artificial sweeteners is that they do not fool the brain. The instant the sweetness receptors on the tongue sense that something sweet is being ingested (that includes most artificial sweeteners), the brain is alerted. In turn, the brain signals the pancreas to begin to release insulin. This "gustatory (or taste-initiated) insulin response" in the absence of any actual caloric intake has the same effect on blood sugar as if a high caloric load were being consumed. Increasing insulin levels drive circulating blood sugar into the cells, where it is converted to glycogen or stored as fat. Blood sugar levels drop and appetite hormones release, prompting more food ingestion. Studies have shown that *individuals who consume artificial sweeteners actually have a greater risk of weight gain and obesity.*

"Sugar-free" honey is another story. This product is not honey at all but an adulterated syrup blend sweetened with maltitol, a sugar alcohol that is a disaccharide (made up of two different sugars). Maltitol has an effect on blood sugar levels similar to sugar, and its caloric load is similar to sucrose. In addition, its larger molecular structure means that it is not absorbed in the upper part of the small intestine like sugar or honey but passes into the large intestine. Here, it is partially metabolized to form triglycerides, or fatty acids, which then contribute to elevated lipids and increased fat deposits throughout the body. Maltitol also produces undesirable digestive tract consequences including excess gas and bloating for many who consume it.

The Dieter's Dilemma and Artificial Sweeteners

Janice, Barb, and Ann worked in the same office. They were all somewhat overweight, constantly dieting it seemed, and all equally unsuccessful in losing weight in spite of constant effort. Each day, they collectively consumed numerous diet soft drinks with the hope of limiting calories and shedding a few pounds. Each month, they found themselves in need of wardrobe expansions.

An office associate suggested that they abandon their diet drinks and start drinking regular soda. Incredulous as it may have seemed, the three agreed to follow the advice, perhaps out of desperation more than common sense.

More incredulous than the advice were the results that began to manifest themselves in a matter of three or four weeks. Each of the three women reported significant weight loss, ranging from 4 to 6 pounds.

Unable to explain the results except for the elimination of diet sodas, their collective experiences reinforced what researchers have known for some time. The regular consumption of artificially sweetened beverages is associated with more weight gain, more fat accumulation around the midsection, elevated fatty acids in the blood, as well as increased risks for obesity and elevated blood lipids.

The reason for this is quite simple: Receptors on the tongue alert the brain that an incoming sweet load is being ingested. (The sweetness receptors on the tongue do not differentiate between artificial and natural sweeteners.) A signal from the brain then triggers the pancreas to release insulin even though no calories are actually being consumed. Insulin drives the existing circulating blood sugar into the cells where it is stored as fat. Thus, dieters who try to avoid calories by drinking diet soft drinks gain weight anyway!

Most artificial sweeteners trigger what we referred to before as the "gustatory insulin response." A precipitous drop in blood sugar from the release of insulin prompts the release of appetite-stimulating hormones, increasing food ingestion and weight gain over time. This is exactly the phenomenon experienced by our three dieters and by countless others who follow their doctor's advice to use artificial sweeteners as a means of limiting calories and losing weight. Better to take a bit of honey and maintain a stable blood sugar than experience the yo-yo effect common to so many dieters who wrongly depend on artificial sweeteners.

Honey: Nature's Amazing Medicine

Honey and Sleep

SLEEP IS AN energy-driven, physiological process. When we retire to bed, our body goes (or should go) to work! This simple statement of scientific fact contradicts much of modern popular thinking regarding what exactly happens during the eight hours of the night fast. This thinking is based on the notion that because no physical exercise occurs, sleep is a process that somehow uses little or no energy. From this we wrongly conclude that eating in the period before bed is not necessary and will result in food being converted into fat and stored in the fat tissue—a myth passed on from generation to generation. Nothing could be further from the scientific truth.

Most of the energy required for the brain, kidneys, and red blood cells during sleep (about 10 grams per hour) must be sourced from the liver. Quality, healthful, restorative sleep is dependent on an adequate stock of liver glycogen, and the liver can only store about 80 grams of glycogen. Therefore, to avoid triggering metabolic stress, the liver glycogen store must be "topped off" before going to bed (see the Liver Depletion Rate graph and note on pages 34-35). When fueled by adequate liver glycogen during the period of the night fast, restorative sleep promotes recovery physiology, and recovery physiology is reparative—a vigorous rebuilding and restorative activity affecting all tissues in the body.

Recovery physiology is also primarily fat-burning physiology, utilizing fat stores for energy requirements. But fat-burning physiology functions at rest only when the brain is provided with an adequate glycogen supply to get through the night. By consciously restocking the liver with honey—the ideal liver/brain food—before bedtime, we activate the HYMN (HoneY-MelatoniN) Cycle.[2] This wonderful metabolic cycle promotes quality, healthful, restorative sleep, and restorative sleep prompts recovery and fat-burning physiology.

Honey is the perfect food to provide energy for the brain during the night fast because it ensures that recovery physiology can continue uninterrupted. The primary reasons for this are simple and straightforward:

- Honey packs a dense caloric load: a small amount provides a relatively large amount of energy.
- Honey presents the gut with a low digestive burden. Absorption into the blood stream is rapid, leaving the GI (gastrointestinal) tract quiet for the night.

---

[2] A complete description of the HYMN Cycle may be found in our book *Smart Sleep: How to Sleep Your Way to Better Health (with Honey)*, WorldClassEmprise, LLC (2010).

- Honey ingestion results in immediate formation of liver glycogen, which fuels the brain during the night fast.

A well-fueled brain is a happy brain, able to orchestrate the events of recovery and restoration during sleep without interruption and without initiating metabolic stress, securing additional energy supplies for itself.

Folks who believe the "Do not eat before bedtime" myth do themselves a great disservice. Sleep is a high-energy enterprise for the brain. Therefore, it is essential that the brain be provided with enough glycogen for fuel to last throughout the eight hours of the night fast. *Fueling the liver with honey before bedtime fuels the brain.*

At all times, but especially during sleep, the brain actively and aggressively defends its energy supply when glucose is scarce. When glucose runs low, as in the early morning hours if the liver was not restocked just before bedtime, the brain activates metabolic stress to ensure its own energy supply.

Metabolic stress is a protective form of adrenal-driven response activated by a signal from the liver that fuel supplies are running low. The adrenal glands respond by releasing adrenalin and cortisol. These "stress hormones" are responsible for the breakdown of the body's protein into amino acids, which are transported to the liver for the formation of new glucose (gluconeogenesis) to provide fuel for the hungry brain.

Energy/glucose homeostasis (regulation) during sleep is a major challenge for most Americans who go to bed without adequate energy stores for the brain to last through the night. Chronic and repeated disruption of sleep by metabolic stress during the night eventually results in impaired glucose regulation and increased insulin resistance.

This is the major cause of metabolic impairments known collectively as the metabolic syndrome. It is the chronic and repeated activation of metabolic stress that results in interrupted or short sleep night after night, for weeks or months, that ultimately results in one or more manifestations of the metabolic syndrome.

The simple strategy of consuming a tablespoon or two of unfiltered honey before bedtime will provide an adequate supply of fuel reserve for the brain throughout the nocturnal fast and ensure that sleep is restful and uninterrupted by metabolic stress. Sleep without stress is conducive for recovery and restoration of body organs, tissues, and immune system functions.

Poor-quality sleep or short sleep is a risk factor in each of the metabolic diseases or conditions discussed in the following sections (beginning on page 35). Honey ingestion before bedtime improves sleep quality and increases the duration of sleep, and thus reduces the risks for these diseases. The fact that honey promotes restorative sleep makes honey a powerful food in preventing disease and restoring health.

Liver Glycogen Depletion Rate in Grams Versus Time

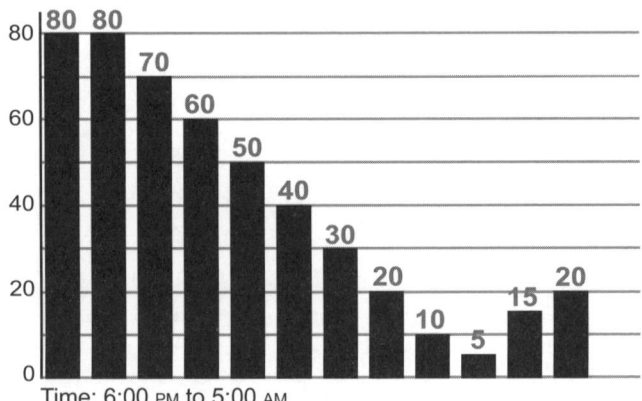

Time: 6:00 PM to 5:00 AM

Note: This graph indicates the levels of liver glycogen following a meal at 6:00 PM. Approximate levels are shown for the next eleven hours, assuming no food intake after 6:00 PM and a normal liver glycogen depletion rate. The total amount of glycogen in the liver at any given time is highly variable. Estimates of total glycogen range from 50 to 120 grams, depending on body size. Liver glycogen depletion rates will also vary depending on activity and demand. At rest, the liver glycogen store will deplete at a rate of about 10 grams per hour, providing 6.5 grams for the brain and 3.5 grams for the kidneys and red blood cells. As liver glycogen levels approach zero, IGFBP-1 (insulin-like growth factor binding protein-1) is released to signal the brain of imminent fuel shortage. The brain responds by triggering metabolic stress, which promotes formation of new glucose (gluconeogenesis).

Honey for Depression

Depression is a multi-factored, complex family of conditions that affect various brain regions in different ways. In advance of actual clinical manifestation of depression, poor-quality and shortened sleep have been shown to be causative factors. Environmental and psychological stresses are also contributors, many of which are difficult to control.

The most significant form of recurrent stress—endogenous or internal metabolic stress—is controllable, and herein lies the greatest hope for those suffering from depression. This form of stress is driven by hunger signals from the brain, or cerebral hunger.

All the modern metabolic diseases, of which depression is one manifestation, may be improved by optimal provision of cerebral energy at critical times during the 24-hour circadian cycle (the biological response to light/dark changes during the day). The key is an optimal and adequate supply of liver glycogen—the only glycogen store that provides glucose to the circulation for brain uptake during the night fast. Honey forms liver glycogen directly. A stable storehouse of liver glycogen eliminates cerebral hunger, reduces metabolic stress, and lowers the risk of metabolic conditions, including depression.

Honey for Diabetes

Honey consumption regulates blood sugar, reducing the highs and preventing the lows, and regular honey consumption results in lower average blood sugar levels (10 to 20 milligrams percent or more) and in lower HbA1c levels (0.2 to 0.4 percent). After ingestion, honey is rapidly absorbed and converted into glycogen in the liver, thus removing glucose from the circulation and lowering blood sugar levels.

The effect of honey on blood sugar levels is due to its ideal combination of fructose and glucose—a unique composition that facilitates the direct formation of liver glycogen and lowers blood sugar levels. Lower blood sugar levels mean a lessened demand for and release of insulin, thus accounting for a stabilization of blood sugar within the circulation.

Honey consumption before bedtime also limits the production and release of cortisol during the night. Cortisol is an adrenal hormone present during rest to ensure that circulating blood sugar levels remain adequate to fuel the brain during sleep. When liver glycogen levels are adequate, cortisol is not needed for this function. A reduction in cortisol levels means that one experiences less metabolic stress and has a lower risk for the diseases and conditions associated with the metabolic syndrome.

Duane's Diabetes and Honey Story

Duane was in his 50s when his doctor diagnosed his diabetes. He wasn't particularly overweight, but a sedentary lifestyle as a pastor and counselor, combined with irregular eating habits, had taken its toll. After his diagnosis, he became "religious" about monitoring his blood sugar levels, sometimes three to four times a day, and keeping accurate records. Modest dietary changes and medication seemed to help control his "numbers," yet over time his blood sugar averages began to creep up again.

Nearing the age of 70, Duane found his blood sugar averages running 10 to 15 milligrams percent higher than his target range, especially in the morning upon awakening. His HbA1c level was acceptable at 6.1 percent, though he wanted to see it lower.

His physician brother-in-law suggested that a tablespoon of honey consumed before bedtime could bring his "numbers" down and boldly predicted that his next HbA1c would be down by 0.2 to 0.4 percent. The advice seemed counterintuitive ("Eating sugar before bedtime to *lower* blood sugar?"), yet he was up for the challenge. Duane began taking honey before retiring for the night.

After three weeks of consistently downing a tablespoon of honey before bed, Duane reported that his morning blood sugar levels were averaging 10 to 15 milligrams percent lower, and his blood sugar averages throughout the day were stabilizing within a normal range. Anticipating his next checkup in a

> month, he was encouraged to stay the course and make no other changes in his diet.
>
> His next doctor's visit confirmed the prediction: Duane's HbA1c report came back at 5.8 percent. Nothing else had changed in his diet or lifestyle routine except for the addition of a tablespoon of honey before bedtime.

Duane's story is not unique. Anecdotal accounts from countless individuals across varying age groups have repeated his story. The simple addition of a tablespoon of honey consumed before bedtime has resulted in the stabilization of blood sugar levels within a normal range. This experience has been consistent without regard to what medication may be taken or the severity of glucose intolerance. In fact, parents of juvenile (type 1) diabetic children have noted less fluctuation in blood sugar levels and less challenge in anticipating insulin demands when they added honey to the treatment regimen. The physicians of these diabetic patients have not been so understanding, however.

Most doctors in the United States do not know that honey is frequently used as the first line of treatment for glucose intolerance for patients in other countries around the world. Most do not recognize that a tablespoon of honey is essentially equivalent in sugar content to a small apple, yet they would not hesitate to recommend fruit in the diet of their diabetic patients.

Honey for Gastrointestinal Health

The influence of stress on gastrointestinal metabolism and health cannot be discounted. Negative stress influences are exerted both centrally from the brain and locally from cells in the digestive tract. What may be more surprising is the increasing clinical evidence that links a distressed GI tract with insomnia and the major mood disorders, such as depression, hypothalamic-pituitary-adrenal (HPA) axis over-activity, and excess secretion of cortisol.

The role of melatonin as a gastro-protective hormone has also been recently confirmed. Activation of sleep and recovery physiology by way of the HYMN Cycle, which promotes melatonin release, is initiated by the ingestion of honey before bed. *This strategy is recommended as a simple and inexpensive way to improve gut physiology and function.* Melatonin opposes the actions of cortisol and serotonin, and both cortisol and serotonin exert destabilizing influences on intestinal physiology when chronically overproduced.

Melatonin is one of the human body's most potent antioxidants. Clinical studies have examined this action of melatonin in gastric ulceration caused by stress, alcohol, anti-inflammatory medications, and H. pylori infection and found melatonin to be protective in gastric lesions as well as a promising therapeutic agent in the control of gastric ulcerations.

In addition to promoting the release of melatonin during sleep, honey ingestion may play a direct role in combating H. pylori infections associated with gastric ulcers. Honey is a powerful antibiotic known to destroy bacteria, including H. pylori, at low concentrations (less than 10 percent). Regular consumption of honey will prove to be an inexpensive and effective method of treating gastric ulceration.

Honey for the Heart

The human heart never sleeps; it must always recover "on the fly." The most potent risk factor for heart disease is chronic exposure to increased levels of the stress hormones cortisol and adrenalin. Chronically increased levels of adrenaline increase heart rate and blood pressure. Chronically elevated cortisol levels cause hypertension, arrhythmia, stroke, and atherosclerosis.

Honey consumption reduces metabolic stress during rest, thus reducing the stress on the heart while it is recovering. Honey also reduces chronic cortisol and adrenalin production and release during the night, thus lowering the risk for cardiovascular disease.

Honey for the Immune System

Optimum functioning of the immune system is profoundly interconnected with other aspects of metabolism and energy homeostasis. Many clinical studies have demonstrated the association between sleep loss and compromised immune function. Other clinical and laboratory studies have demonstrated that regular consumption of honey results in elevation of platelet counts, stabilization of hemoglobin levels, and improvements in white blood cell counts—all results that are associated with improved immune system functioning.

The provision of an adequate and sustained cerebral energy supply during the period of nocturnal fasting promotes restorative sleep and improved immune system functioning, and the ingestion of honey before bedtime makes this possible.

Honey for Melatonin and the Mind

Research over the last two decades suggests that melatonin is critical in memory and learning. Its role in memory consolidation and learning in cerebral metabolism may indeed be its most important. Some researchers now regard melatonin as the *learning hormone*.

Melatonin is a hormone with a wide range of beneficial actions: It is a potent antioxidant; it reduces stress by inhibiting cortisol and adrenaline release; it exhibits anti-aging potential; it promotes quality sleep and recovery physiology; it exhibits neuro-protective and anti-carcinogenic properties; and it relieves anxiety.

Given the fact that quality sleep is critical to memory consolidation and human learning, it would seem logical to conclude that optimizing recovery physiology by reducing chronic overproduction of adrenal stress hormones (which inhibit melatonin) and maximizing the production and release of melatonin would be a sound investment in promoting the health of the brain. The only practical way that this may be achieved, however, is by optimally replenishing liver glycogen stores in the period before sleep. And the "gold standard" food for this purpose is pure, unfiltered honey. This strategy produces the exact metabolic environment required to allow for the release of melatonin, growth hormone, and IGF-1—the key hormones of memory consolidation and learning.

Honey for Menopause and Infertility

Several research studies conducted within the last ten years have presented evidence of the strong links between adrenal- (or cortisol-) driven stress, menstrual irregularities, and both male and female infertility. These findings provide a direct link to the metabolic syndrome and the spectrum of modern metabolic-stress-driven conditions.

The simple nostrum of an ounce of quality honey ingested each night before bedtime is an inexpensive and risk-free strategy to control internal metabolic stress. By so doing, one selectively restocks the liver glycogen store for the night fast, ensures adequate provisions for the brain, and facilitates recovery physiology. The consequent reduction in adrenal stress hormones from the reduction or elimination of chronic metabolic stress ultimately improves reproductive health and facilitates optimal fertility.

Honey for Sleep Disorders

Obstructive sleep apnea (OSA), or sleep apnea, is a condition of interrupted breathing during sleep that reduces oxygen delivery to the brain and creates a "reflex" arousal and interruption of sleep. The cycle often continues throughout the night, resulting in significant sleep loss, fatigue, and excessive daytime sleepiness the following day. Sleep apnea increases the risk for all the diseases known collectively as the metabolic syndrome: heart disease, diabetes, obesity. The increased risk is the result of chronic increased nocturnal stress and inflammation every night in life.

Sleep apnea is emerging as a consistent common link among a growing list of diseases caused by poor-quality sleep and chronic stress overnight—a list that includes a wide range of diseases such as depression and Alzheimer's disease. The only way to reduce this overnight stress and reduce these risks is to provision the brain with a sufficient fuel supply from the liver prior to bedtime. The best way to do this is by the ingestion of an ounce or two of quality, unfiltered honey. Honey activates the HYMN Cycle, which initiates restorative sleep and promotes recovery physiology. Additionally, the production and release of adrenal stress hormones is reduced, allowing sleep to continue uninterrupted throughout the night.

Honey for Thyroid Conditions

Normal functioning of the thyroid gland can be disrupted by chronic partial nocturnal fasting, chronic partial sleep deprivation, and chronic nocturnal metabolic stress—the three toxic strands of modern lifestyle. Recent medical studies have shown a strong association between the adrenal stress hormones (cortisol and adrenalin) released in these conditions and impairments in thyroid function, especially hypothyroidism or low thyroid function. Many direct and indirect links exist between the thyroid and the HPA (hypothalamic-pituitary-adrenal, or stress) axis as evidenced by significant negative associated influences. Low thyroid function is also known to be a risk for cardiovascular disease, obesity, osteoporosis, Alzheimer's disease, and memory loss in the aging.

The above conditions are related to the development of the metabolic syndrome, which is intimately related to chronic nocturnal metabolic stress. Again, the simple strategy of restocking the liver glycogen store with honey before bedtime plays a role in the modulation and/or elimination of metabolic stress.

Honey and Dreams

The most common and interesting anecdotes reported from those who consume a tablespoon or two of honey before bedtime relate to dreams and dream recall. Dreams are more vivid, intense, and colorful. The reports have become so frequent that conclusive opinions are merited.

Dreams are known to occur during the rapid eye movement (REM) portion of sleep. The ingestion of honey before bedtime provides sufficient fuel for the brain so that REM sleep ("dream sleep") occurs in its normal cycles, uninterrupted by metabolic stress. Direct association between improvements in REM sleep and honey consumption will have to await confirmation from studies that are underway.

However, it is known that honey improves memory and reduces anxiety when compared to sucrose. Honey also reduces metabolic and oxidative stress, both of which affect the duration and quality of sleep.

The hypothesis that honey eaten before bedtime increases REM sleep and therefore improves memory processing presents us with a model for improved learning. Logic supports the fact that liver (glycogen) replenishment prior to bedtime ensures restorative sleep and increases REM sleep, both of which facilitate offline processing, memory consolidation, and learning. More research is needed to confirm this simple hypothesis. In the meantime, *there is no risk associated with consuming honey before bedtime*. Those who have begun this habit may find themselves well ahead of the game in experiencing improved brain function.

Honey and Alzheimer's Disease

It is now recognized that the complex set of conditions known as the metabolic syndrome includes not only obesity and type 2 diabetes but other conditions driven by internal metabolic stress, such as sleep disorders and neuro-degenerative diseases like Alzheimer's and Parkinson's. Type 2 diabetes is a major health concern in Western society, affecting more than 27 million (nearly 10 percent of the population in the United States).

A growing consensus is pointing to the conclusion that not only are the neuro-degenerative diseases associated with diabetes, but they represent a specialized type of diabetes that afflicts various regions of the brain with differing outcomes. These conditions are, in effect, a manifestation of "cerebral diabetes" in that they mirror in the brain the breakdown in energy management and disposal that occurs in the body with classic type 2 diabetes. Some have called this type 3 diabetes.

The link between internal metabolic stress, chronic nocturnal stress, and abnormal sleep patterns has been described previously. Sleep apnea follows this pattern of metabolic impairments. Sleep apnea has also been linked by a specific gene to Alzheimer's disease, and this gene is also linked to heart disease.

While the association between chronic nocturnal stress and interrupted sleep patterns is consistent with reason, the finding that there is a genetic link between sleep apnea and Alzheimer's disease is more of a surprise. This connection would suggest that an improvement in sleep patterns in the elderly may significantly lessen the manifestation and progression of the disease. The provision of a dose of quality honey before bedtime should be one essential aspect of treatment. Honey will then improve recovery physiology and improve memory consolidation and retrieval as it activates the HYMN Cycle.

Honey and Aging

Some would argue that the afflictions of aging cannot be prevented, or that it is too late for prevention; treatment is the only option. That belief is illustrated by the increasing number of prescriptive medicines taken every day by the elderly. The unfortunate fact is that it may be too late for preventive strategies for some. Lifelong habits of dietary abuses and lifestyle choices have reaped certain rewards.

However, for many, perhaps the great majority, the following suggestions (or "directives") can be put in place today that will produce months and years of healthy life. They carry no risk, produce no side effects, are drug free, and cost but pennies a day. And while they may not cure all of one's diseases, their implementation will bring about positive changes in one's health in a matter of days or weeks, regardless of age.

Directives for Better Health

1. **Don't go to bed hungry**! Avoidance of food in the hours before bedtime ensures certain metabolic disaster during the nocturnal fast.

2. **Give your liver a chance to make and store glycogen not only before bedtime but throughout the day.** (Adequate liver glycogen formation will not come from continuing to consume excessive amounts of sugar and high-fructose corn syrup.) Avoid liver depletion!

3. **Eliminate excess sucrose and HFCS from your diet.** These foods (and processed foods that contain them) only raise blood sugar levels and produce hyperinsulinemia (excessive insulin secretion). Excess glucose and fructose get stored as fat.

4. **Keep your brain happy by providing it with fuel first.** When the brain is happy, the whole body is happy! Remember that the brain depends primarily on liver glycogen for fuel, and a well-fueled brain prevents metabolic stress.

5. **Adopt a simple strategy of consuming unfiltered honey every day**: a tablespoon or more at bedtime, a tablespoon in the morning with breakfast, and one or two during the day before and after periods of exercise.

These simple suggestions will result in one or more of the following benefits:

1. You will sleep better and longer, as the insomnia caused by metabolic stress will be eliminated. Restorative sleep will be enhanced and recovery physiology will occur without interruption throughout the night.

2. Your sleep patterns will include more frequent periods of REM sleep. Your dreams will be more vivid and your dream recall remarkable.
3. Your memory consolidation and recall will improve.
4. Your blood sugar levels will stabilize (the highs and lows will be eliminated), and your food cravings will gradually go away. (If you are diabetic, your HbA1c levels will decrease.)
5. You will awaken in the morning feeling more rested and without feelings of intense hunger, shakiness, nausea, or weakness.
6. Your total cholesterol and triglyceride levels will come down, and your HDL (high-density lipoproteins, or "good") cholesterol level will increase gradually.
7. You may lose a little weight, but perhaps more importantly, you will burn more body fat during the night to fuel the normal recovery and restoration of body tissues that occur during rest.
8. The inflammatory processes that accompany aging will become less intense and symptomatic. Risk factors for all of the diseases of aging that are associated with chronic inflammation will gradually be reduced.

Honey: The Superfuel for Exercise

DURING EXERCISE, ENERGY stores are being rapidly depleted as if in a state of aggressive starvation. If those energy stores are not rapidly replenished, the body must mobilize all resources to maintain the level of physical output while maintaining all essential metabolic activity. In particular, a fuel supply for the brain must be provided.

When exercising, the brain must be fueled exclusively from the liver glycogen store, while contracting muscles may be fueled from both muscle glycogen and liver glycogen. An early warning fuel detection system is essential so that the liver may warn the brain of an impending fuel shortage. Beginning with the onset of exercise and throughout the exercise duration, the liver signals the brain when its fuel store is running low. This results in an inhibition of another signaling protein that drives glucose into muscles. When this occurs, less glucose is taken in by contracting muscles, thus keeping more glucose in circulation to fuel the brain. However, the tradeoff is that less glucose oxidation takes place within muscle cells at a significant reduction in power output.

The Five Critical Times for Fueling for Exercise

There are five times during a 24-hour day that are critical for proper exercise fueling:

- Upon arising
- Before exercise
- During exercise
- Post exercise
- Before recovery sleep

In the early morning hours or upon awakening, the liver requires attention. Glycogen stores are nearly depleted after eight hours of sleep, assuming one retired with a fully stocked liver. The brain, if it has not begun to do so already, is responding to the signal from the liver and is correctly sensing that its fuel supply is low. Fueling before and during exercise are both equally important so that liver glycogen stores are adequately maintained and unnecessary metabolic stress is prevented.

The post-exercise refueling period must also give attention to replenishing the liver glycogen stores. This will occur if one includes some fructose-containing foods, such as fruits and vegetables or *honey*, which ensure that the liver takes in and stores glucose. However, any liver glycogen formed will be quickly released from the liver during this period to provide glucose for depleted muscle tissue. Therefore it is also recommended to do some selective refueling of the liver in the post-exercise period before bedtime, when recovery physiology is the key metabolic consideration.

The importance of proper fueling during training and competition is again underscored. Strategies that fuel the liver before, during, and post exercise must be directed at securing and maintaining liver glycogen stores and protecting against protein catabolism. To disregard this critical fact places the athlete at risk of a host of metabolic conditions that directly result from protein loss due to metabolic stress.

Don't Be Confused About Energy

There are many "energy drinks" and "energy boosters" on the market these days, and most of them promise to "release energy." Remember, there is a difference between releasing energy and *providing* energy. Many substances will release energy into the blood stream; caffeine is the best example of this. But caffeine is a thermogenic (heat-producing) drug: it increases the metabolic rate and prompts the release of fatty acids into the blood stream. Unfortunately, most of these fatty acids return to the fat stores after exercise and contribute little to energy requirements.

The primary energy source used by the body for exercise is glucose, and the more intense the level of exercise, the higher percentage of glucose to fat is burned. The best possible "energy-providing" food is honey. Not only does honey provide the correct balance of fructose to glucose, but it will also optimally and selectively refuel the liver without a significant digestive burden during post-exercise recovery. This is an important consideration, as digestion is a metabolically expensive and energy-demanding series of physiologic processes.

The amount of honey necessary after exercise and before rest periods will vary according to body size and the status of liver glycogen stores. Typically, one or two tablespoons provides optimum fuel to ensure adequate liver glycogen during recovery times. And when adequate liver glycogen stores are available during rest, fat burning will be optimized during that time.

Honey is the highest-octane natural fuel available to humans for exercise and recovery!

Ten Basic Facts for Exercise Fueling

1. The primary fuel for exercise in humans is glucose, a simple carbohydrate.
2. The greater the intensity of exercise, the higher the percentage of glucose burned relative to fat.
3. The most significant energy storehouse for exercise and recovery is the liver glycogen store.
4. Fueling for muscles and liver should be undertaken before, during, and after exercise, and with respect to the liver, prior to recovery sleep.
5. Fructose is the sugar specifically selected by the liver to facilitate and regulate glucose uptake.
6. A fructose-based fuel (like fruit or *honey*) during exercise will increase oxidation and therefore power output during exercise.

7. Optimal fueling of both the muscles and the liver will reduce production of adrenal stress hormones and protect muscle proteins from degradation.

8. Optimal fueling is as important during training as it is for competition. In one sense it is more important, because it is the daily metabolic toll during training that will impact the athlete's health over his/her competitive life, both in the short and long term.

9. Fats are never a limiting factor during exercise; they are abundantly available. Any attempt to release extra fats during exercise will be counterproductive and promote long-term negative consequences.

10. Proteins may be a significant fuel used during exercise, but good fueling protocols must take the liver into account. The liver glycogen storehouse is critical.

Honey: The All-Star Superfood

Another "Believer" Joined the Revolution

(As told by co-author Dr. Fessenden)

As a woman stepped to the microphone following a recent presentation on "The Effects of Honey on Human Metabolism" at a beekeepers convention in Saskatchewan, I wondered briefly what might be coming from this somewhat overweight individual. She began by saying, "I have joined the honey revolution!"

In surprised and curious silence, I waited for her to continue.

"Six months ago I was very much overweight, much more so than now. I had borderline diabetes, and my doctor was considering what interventions may be necessary for my elevated blood sugar and cholesterol. I couldn't sleep more than three or four hours a night without waking up hungry. Sometimes it took me an hour to get back to sleep. I had purchased your book *The Honey Revolution* a year ago, and I decided that it was the time to see if your advice would work."

She paused briefly and started again, "I am happy to report that I have lost a lot of weight, and my blood sugar and cholesterol levels are normal. My doctor was happy and I was thrilled, but more importantly . . . "

What could be better than what she had already reported? I thought.

Then she continued, "I sleep through the night without interruption. I wake up feeling rested. I haven't felt this good in my life! Thank you for your book, and thank God for honey!"

Of all the responses from individuals who have reported their experiences after starting to consume a small amount of honey before bedtime, the "Another 'Believer'" testimonial may be the most gratifying. It is also the most common response reported by almost three-fourths of those who take the time to email or call or share their stories at conferences.

Improvement in quality and duration of sleep is truly an astounding and revolutionary benefit from the consumption of a bit of honey before bedtime. Surprisingly, this simple intervention has produced amazing results.

"You've changed my life!" is the way one woman from our church choir puts it. (She received a copy of *The Honey Revolution* from a friend.) The fact that honey improves sleep, both in duration and quality, is evidence of its ability to produce liver glycogen directly after ingestion. A full store of liver glycogen at bedtime insures adequate fuel for the brain during the night fast and avoids the onset of metabolic (adrenal-driven) stress during the early morning hours.

The anecdotal reports of vivid dreams and increased dream recall from many are proof of an increase in REM sleep. REM sleep frequency and duration decreases with the aging process, but honey consumption at bedtime appears to reverse this trend.

Not everyone who consumes honey at bedtime will lose weight, but many do. Some report that the simple addition of a tablespoon of honey taken at bedtime is the only thing to which they can attribute the loss of several pounds over a few months. One couple reported a combined 85-pound weight loss over a period of six months! These stories are also consistent with animal studies that show weight loss as a common result of being fed a diet based on honey rather than sucrose or HFCS.

How Much Honey Is Enough

The optimum recommended daily consumption of honey is 3 to 5 tablespoons taken in divided doses. This equates to approximately 54 to 90 grams per day, providing about 200 to 360 calories. Compare that to the average daily consumption of HFCS for every person above age two that is now estimated to be in excess of 330 to 800 grams, or 1320 to 3200 calories, per day!

For best results, 1 to 2 tablespoons of honey should be consumed just before bedtime. Another tablespoon should be consumed with breakfast in the morning, and another tablespoon or two is recommended before and after any period of exercise during the day.

Remember to buy only raw, unfiltered honey, preferably from packers or honey producers that you know.[3]

Know your beekeeper, know your honey.
And for your good health, enjoy honey and
join the honey revolution!

---

[3] This statement simply indicates that the studies on which this book's health benefits are derived have been based exclusively on the consumption of raw, unfiltered honey. It is not meant to imply that the processed honey packed and sold under several well-known brand names is bad for you.

Frequently Asked Questions

THE SECTION PRESENTS information contained in this book in a simple question-and-answer format edited for the average reader. References and citations for the facts contained herein may be found in the unabridged versions of *The Honey Revolution* and *Smart Sleep*.

Q: *What is honey?*

A: Honey is a natural, sweet substance, made from the nectar of flowering plants and trees by honeybees, to which nothing has been added and nothing taken away. It is composed of nearly equal proportions of the simple sugars fructose and glucose, plus small amounts of other sugars, and is about 18 percent water.

Over 180 different substances have been identified in honey, including 5 enzymes, 6 vitamins, 8 lipids, trace amounts of 12 minerals and 17 elements, 18 different acids, 18 amino acids (proteins), 18 bioflavonoids, and 26 aroma compounds. Currently, there are more than 300 varietals of honey produced in the United States.

Q: How many calories are there in a tablespoon of honey?

A: One tablespoon (21 grams) of honey provides 64 calories, primarily from carbohydrates or sugars.

Q: If half of the sugar found in honey is fructose, isn't that a lot? Isn't fructose supposed to be bad for you?

A: Fructose, also known as "fruit sugar," is not harmful to your health if consumed in the small amounts typically found in fruits, most vegetables, and honey. Each tablespoon of honey contains about 8 grams of fructose on average, the same amount found in one small apple. Fructose is essential for the liver to create and store glucose as glycogen.

Q: So, what's the problem with fructose that I keep hearing about?

A: The major problem with fructose is the amount that is consumed each day. The average American, above the age of two, consumes 330 grams (0.73 pounds) of high-fructose corn syrup (HFCS), which contains 55 percent fructose or 182 grams each day. That much fructose simply overwhelms the liver, which is the main place in the body where fructose can be metabolized. Some fructose gets converted to glucose in the liver and stored as glycogen. When confronted with more fructose than it can handle, the liver stops everything else that it is doing to break down the fructose into three carbon molecules. These then get converted into fatty acids and released into the circulation to be carried to fat tissue throughout the body and stored as fat. This amount of fructose consumption is the main reason we have an epidemic of obesity in the United States.

Q: *How does the fructose in honey help the liver store glucose?*

A: Fructose unlocks the enzyme hidden in the liver cell nuclei that is necessary to convert glucose to glycogen. (This enzyme is called glucokinase.) When fructose and glucose are present together, fructose assists the liver in taking glucose out of the circulation. This effectively lowers blood sugar by removing glucose from the blood stream and bringing it into the liver, where it is converted to glycogen and stored.

Without fructose, glucose passes through the liver and into the blood, triggering the release of insulin. Insulin drives glucose into the cells where it is used as energy or stored as fat.

Q: *Is there a difference between glucose stored in the muscle cells as glycogen and the glycogen stored in the liver?*

A: Both muscle glycogen and liver glycogen are multiple glucose molecules joined together into chains. There is a big difference between the two in how they get used in the body. Once glucose enters the muscle cells, it does not come out. Muscle cells trap it there for later use or convert it to fat. Liver glycogen, on the other hand, can be easily converted back to glucose and shared with other cells and organs of the body when needed for energy, especially the red blood cells, the kidneys, and the brain.

Q: Why is it important to maintain a reserve of glycogen in the liver?

A: Liver glycogen is the primary source of fuel reserve for the brain. During sleep and during exercise, the brain is at risk of running out of fuel. During both of those times, the liver glycogen store provides fuel for the brain's energy needs. Without adequate liver glycogen, the brain initiates a form of metabolic stress to provide fuel for itself.

Q: How much glycogen can the liver store?

A: The liver can only store about 75 grams of glycogen at any one time. In some individuals, the liver capacity for glycogen may be as low as 50 grams or as high as 120 grams. The exact capacity of the liver glycogen store is difficult to measure directly but may be estimated by other indicators.

Q: How much glycogen does the liver release as glucose for the body during rest?

A: At rest, the liver releases 10 grams of glucose per hour: 6.5 grams for the brain, and 3.5 grams for the kidneys and red blood cells. That means that the brain only has enough glucose from the liver for about seven to eight hours.

Q: How much glycogen is released from the liver during exercise?

A: During exercise, the liver may release glucose at a rate of up to 100 grams per hour, depending on the intensity of the exercise. That means that the brain can survive for about 45 minutes until it needs to refuel.

Q: *Does the brain have any other source of fuel?*

A: Yes. The brain will burn some amino acids from proteins. After several days of starvation, the brain will also begin to burn ketones (organic compounds) derived from fats. However, the primary source of fuel for the brain is glucose from the blood and from the liver. The brain cells contain only enough fuel to survive about 30 seconds, and there is enough glucose in the blood (blood sugar) at any one time for the brain to survive about 30 minutes.

Q: *What happens when the brain runs out of fuel?*

A: If that were to happen, one would lapse into a coma and eventually die. But the brain protects itself so that it will not run out of fuel. It does this by initiating a form of metabolic stress.

Q: *What is metabolic stress?*

A: Metabolic stress is a protective mechanism initiated by the brain when it senses its fuel reserve in the liver is running low—sort of like the "low fuel" light coming on in your car when the gas tank is nearly empty. When this happens, the brain triggers the adrenal glands to release adrenalin and cortisol. These hormones then mobilize alternative fuel stores, such as fatty acids and protein from muscle tissue. The protein from muscle tissue gets broken down into amino acids that are carried back to the liver, where they are converted to new glucose for the brain. Metabolic stress is sometimes referred to as the "fight or flight" reaction. The intent is to protect the fuel supply for the brain.

Q: Does metabolic stress ever occur at night as we sleep?

A: Absolutely and frequently for many of us. When we go to bed without replenishing our liver glycogen store, there may only be enough glycogen supply in the liver to fuel the brain for 4 to 5 hours.

Q: What does metabolic stress do if it happens during sleep?

A: It does the same thing as when it happens during waking hours: adrenalin and cortisol are released. Adrenalin raises our heart rate and blood pressure and wakes us up; cortisol triggers a host of other changes in our resting physiology that preserve and create an adequate glucose supply for the brain. The end result is that our sleep is interrupted until the brain is assured of having a sufficient fuel supply to allow sleep to continue.

Q: Does consuming honey before bedtime prevent metabolic stress from happening?

A: Yes, indeed! Honey, with its ideal ratio of fructose to glucose, allows for immediate glycogen formation in the liver ("tops off the tank"). When the liver glycogen store is full, the brain has enough fuel to get through the night without interruption. Honey "energizes" the brain for rest.

Q: Will eating other foods prevent metabolic stress also?

A: Yes, but with consequences. A small portion of fruit (about 1 cup) contains about the same amount of fructose and glucose as 1 tablespoon of honey. A small serving of most vegetables also contains similar amounts of glucose and fructose.

However, eating fruits and vegetables before bedtime adds to the work of the digestive tract at a time when the activity there is being "powered down" in preparation for rest. Vegetables also contain a large amount of starch, another carbohydrate, which is immediately converted to glucose in our stomach and small intestine. As it enters the blood stream, this glucose causes a big release of insulin, which drives glucose into the muscle cells and removes it from circulation, keeping it from the brain. Within a couple of hours, our blood sugar level falls and causes metabolic stress. A small amount of honey (1 to 2 tablespoons) is the best food with which to restock the liver glycogen store before bed.

Q: *Won't honey raise my blood sugar also?*

A: A small dose of honey does not raise blood sugar as much as an equivalent dose of glucose or sugar (sucrose); it does not trigger a large insulin spike. Honey controls or regulates blood sugar and helps to stabilize it within a normal range.

Q: *Does honey do anything else to help me sleep?*

A: Yes. The glucose portion of honey does trigger a small insulin release. Insulin in the blood causes a substance called tryptophan to be driven into the brain, where it is converted to serotonin. Serotonin promotes relaxation. In total darkness, serotonin is converted to melatonin, which then activates sleep. This is what we call the HoneY-MelatoniN (HYMN) Cycle and describe in detail in our upcoming book, *Smart Sleep: How to Sleep Your Way to Better Health (with Honey)*.

Q: *You said earlier that honey "energizes" my brain for rest. I thought my brain needed to sleep, not be energized during rest. What about that?*

A: Sleep is actually a high-energy state for the brain. During sleep, the brain requires as much fuel as when it is awake (some researchers even say it needs more). When you go to sleep, your brain goes to work. Providing energy for the brain during rest allows it to accomplish or control the normal functions of recovery, memory consolidation and learning, immune system improvements, and other benefits of restorative sleep. Without sufficient fuel reserves for the eight hours of rest, sleep will be interrupted, and metabolic stress will be initiated by the brain to ensure adequate fuel for itself.

Q: *Can you describe two significant things that regular honey consumption will do?*

A: Certainly! First, eating honey on a regular basis (3 to 5 tablespoons a day) helps to regulate blood sugar within a normal range and produce and store the liver glycogen needed to fuel the brain. Second, eating a tablespoon of honey before bedtime will result in quality sleep that promotes the occurrence of recovery physiology during the nighttime and eliminates the need for the brain to activate metabolic stress.

Q: *What will eating honey do for all the conditions and diseases related to metabolic stress?*

A: The fact that honey helps to prevent metabolic stress by providing fuel for the brain means that it will also reduce the risks for the conditions and diseases associated with the metabolic syndrome, including obesity, diabetes, hypertension, thyroid conditions, and others described in this book.

Q: *Does honey prevent metabolic stress for everyone?*

A: The principles of how honey is metabolized, forms liver glycogen directly, fuels the brain, and reduces metabolic stress are the same for everyone. However, each person's metabolism is a bit different and is subject to individual, environmental, and genetic factors that may modify or limit the effects of honey consumption. The good news is that the consumption of honey in small amounts daily has no side affects, comes with no risks, and may be safely tried by anyone with a mature immune system (infants over 12 months of age).

Q: *How long will it take for me to experience the effects of honey?*

A: Within a few days, sleep patterns will change and dreams will be more vivid, indicating more restful sleep. And within two to three weeks, blood sugar levels will be more regulated, which will be more obvious to some who are used to experiencing extreme high and low levels.

REFERENCES

REFERENCES FOR THE health benefits afforded by the consumption of honey described in this short book can be found in the following three books from WorldClassEmprise, LLC, by Ron Fessenden, MD, MPH, and Mike McInnes, MRPS:

- *The Hibernation Diet*
  (U.S. edition, WorldClassEmprise, LLC, 2007)
- *The Honey Revolution*
  (WorldClassEmprise, LLC, 2008)
- *Smart Sleep: How to Sleep Your Way to Better Health (with Honey)*, scheduled for publication in 2010 (WorldClassEmprise, LLC)

For more information go to:

www.thehoneyrevolution.com

www.revhoney.com

Or email: info@worldclassemprise.com

ABOUT THE AUTHORS

RON FESSENDEN, MD, MPH, is a retired medical doctor. Dr. Fessenden received his MD degree from the University of Kansas School of Medicine in 1970 and his Masters in Public Health from the University of Hawaii School of Public Health in 1982. For the past three years, he has been researching and writing about the health benefits of honey.

Dr. Fessenden is the co-chairman for the Committee for the Promotion of Honey and Health, Inc., an international organization committed to communicating the message of honey and health, encouraging research on honey, and establishing quality standards for honey worldwide.

MIKE MCINNES, MRPS, is the author of the first edition of *The Hibernation Diet* (Souvenir Press, Ltd.), published in 2006. Mike is a Member of the Royal Pharmaceutical Society of the United Kingdom, and he and his wife, Theresa, and their son, Stuart, founded ISO Active, LTD, in Edinburgh, Scotland, in 1997. ISO Active specializes in a nutritional approach to health and exercise.

Mike has spent twelve years researching and refining his knowledge of the liver physiology and function that formed the basis for *The Hibernation Diet*. This knowledge base has been expanded in *The Honey Revolution* (WorldClassEmprise, LLC) following Mike's participation as a speaker at The First International Symposium on Honey and Human Health, held in Sacramento, California, in January 2008.